LEAKY GUT COOKBOOK

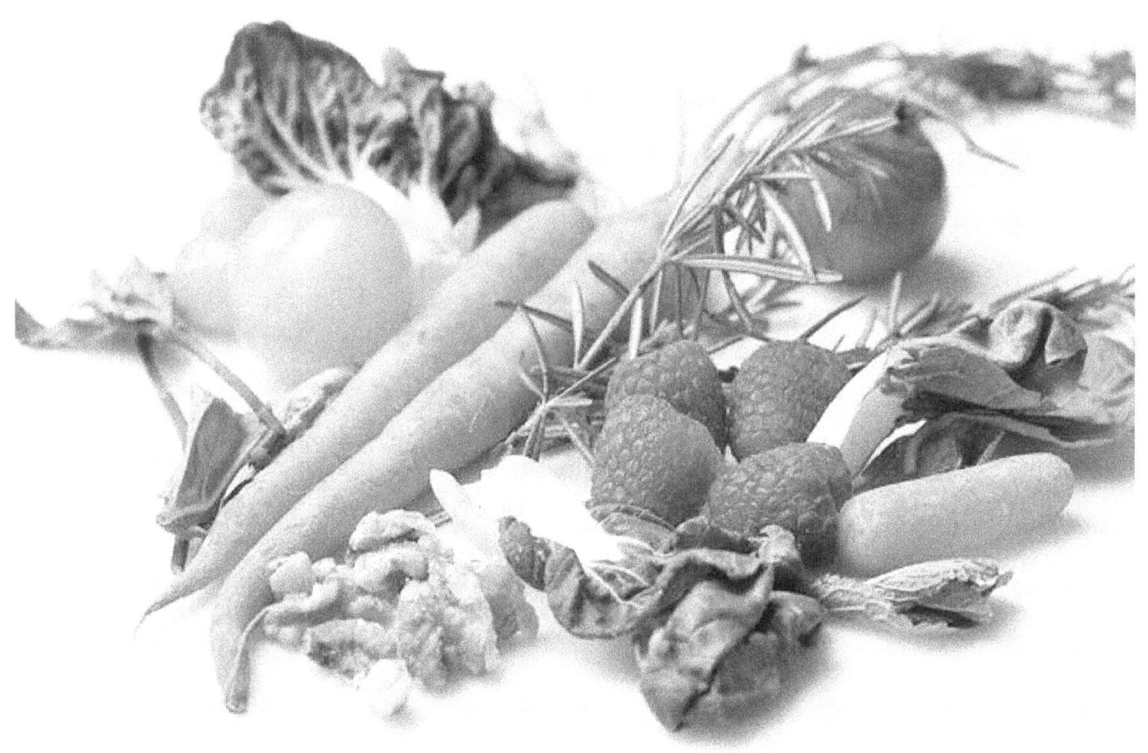

DR. VICKIE STOCK

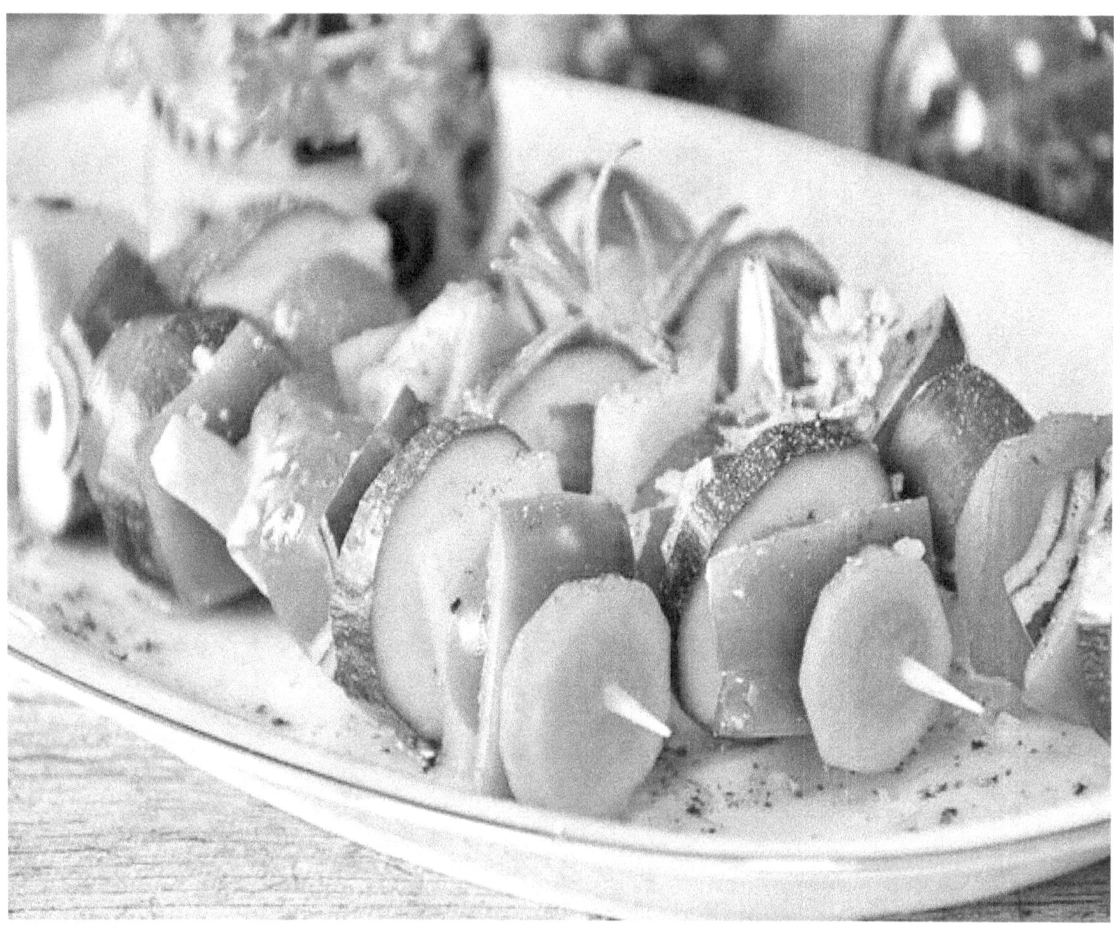

TABLE OF CONTENT

CHAPTER ONE

INTRODUCTION

Leaky Gut Syndrome is a health condition that centers around the permeability of the intestinal lining, creating a breach in the body's natural defense mechanisms. At its essence, the gastrointestinal tract serves as a critical interface between the external environment and the internal workings of the body. In the case of Leaky Gut, this interface becomes compromised, allowing substances that would typically remain within the intestines to pass through into the bloodstream.

The gut lining, comprised of a delicate tapestry of epithelial cells, plays a pivotal role in maintaining a selective barrier. Tight junctions between these cells act as gatekeepers, regulating the passage of nutrients while preventing the entry of potentially harmful particles. When these tight junctions malfunction, the gut becomes "leaky," permitting the uncontrolled flow of undigested food, toxins, and bacteria into the bloodstream.

Several factors contribute to the development of Leaky Gut Syndrome. Poor dietary choices, chronic stress, medications, and environmental factors can all play a role in disrupting the delicate balance of the gut lining. Over time, this disruption can lead to a cascade of inflammatory responses, potentially giving rise to a range of health issues.

Recognizing Leaky Gut Syndrome is challenging due to its diverse and often nonspecific symptoms. Digestive disturbances, food sensitivities, joint pain, and skin conditions may signal the presence of this condition. Diagnosis typically involves a comprehensive assessment of medical history, symptoms, and laboratory tests to gauge inflammation and overall gut health.

In essence, Leaky Gut Syndrome underscores the interconnectedness of gut health with overall well-being. Addressing the root causes, adopting a gut-friendly lifestyle, and seeking guidance from healthcare professionals are essential steps toward restoring balance to the intricate tapestry of the digestive system.

The Anatomy of the Gut

To comprehend Leaky Gut Syndrome, one must first understand the intricate anatomy of the digestive system.

The gastrointestinal tract, a marvelously designed tapestry of organs, plays a crucial role in nutrient absorption, immune function, and maintaining a delicate balance within the body.

The gut lining, consisting of a single layer of epithelial cells, acts as a barrier between the contents of the intestines and the bloodstream. This barrier is selectively permeable, allowing essential nutrients to pass through while blocking the entry of harmful substances.

The Underlying Mechanisms

Leaky Gut Syndrome occurs when the integrity of this protective barrier is compromised. Various factors contribute to this breach, including:

Dysregulation of Tight Junctions: Tight junctions are protein structures that bind adjacent cells together, forming a barrier in the intestinal lining. Disruption of these junctions can lead to increased permeability.

Imbalance in Gut Microbiota: The gut is home to trillions of microorganisms collectively known as the microbiota. An imbalance in this microbial community, often referred to as dysbiosis, can contribute to inflammation and compromise the integrity of the gut lining.

Inflammatory Responses: Chronic inflammation within the gastrointestinal tract can damage the epithelial cells and disrupt the normal functioning of the gut barrier.

Identifying the Culprits

Several factors contribute to the development of Leaky Gut Syndrome. These may include:

Poor Diet: Consuming a diet high in processed foods, refined sugars, and lacking in fiber can contribute to inflammation and negatively impact gut health.

Stress: Chronic stress has been linked to changes in gut permeability, possibly through the release of stress hormones that affect the gut lining.

Medications: Some medications, such as nonsteroidal anti-inflammatory drugs (NSAIDs) and antibiotics, can disrupt the balance of gut bacteria and contribute to increased permeability. Environmental Factors: Exposure to environmental toxins, pollutants, and certain food additives may also play a role in compromising gut integrity.

Managing Leaky Gut Syndrome typically involves a multifaceted approach aimed at addressing the underlying causes and promoting gut healing. Key components of a therapeutic strategy may include:

Dietary Changes: Adopting an anti-inflammatory diet that eliminates trigger foods and emphasizes nutrient-dense, whole foods can play a crucial role in supporting gut health.

Probiotics and Prebiotics: Introducing beneficial bacteria through probiotic supplements and promoting their growth with prebiotic-rich foods can help restore a healthy balance in the gut microbiota.

Supplements: Certain supplements, such as glutamine, zinc, and omega-3 fatty acids, may support gut repair and reduce inflammation.

Stress Management: Incorporating stress-reduction techniques such as mindfulness, meditation, and adequate sleep can positively impact gut health.

Medication Adjustment: Working closely with healthcare providers to assess and potentially adjust medication regimens that may contribute to gut issues.

Leaky Gut Syndrome is a condition with far-reaching implications for overall health. While the intricacies of the gut may seem like a complex tapestry, understanding the fundamentals of this syndrome empowers individuals to take proactive steps toward healing. By addressing contributing factors, adopting a gut-friendly lifestyle, and seeking guidance from healthcare professionals, individuals can embark on a journey towards restoring balance and vitality to their digestive system.

What is Leaky Gut?

Leaky Gut Syndrome, a term that has garnered increasing attention in both medical and wellness circles, refers to a condition where the lining of the intestines becomes more permeable than usual. To comprehend the intricacies of Leaky Gut, one must delve into the fascinating realm of the gastrointestinal tract and the physiological tapestry that constitutes the gut.

The Basics of Leaky Gut

At its core, the gut serves as a complex barrier between the external environment and the internal workings of the body. Imagine the gut lining as a protective fortress, composed of a single layer of epithelial cells tightly knit together. This lining acts as a guardian, allowing essential nutrients to pass through while preventing the entry of harmful substances, toxins, and undigested food particles.

Leaky Gut Syndrome disrupts this delicate balance, causing the junctions between the epithelial cells to loosen. In a healthy gut, these junctions, aptly named tight junctions, form a formidable defense against unwanted invaders. However, in the case of Leaky Gut, these junctions become compromised, leading to an increased permeability that permits the passage of normally restricted substances into the bloodstream.

Causes and Risk factors

Understanding the causes and risk factors associated with Leaky Gut Syndrome provides crucial insights into the intricate web of factors contributing to this condition. While the gut's physiology is remarkably resilient, various influences can compromise its integrity, leading to increased permeability and the onset of Leaky Gut.

Dietary Choices:

Diet plays a pivotal role in the health of the gastrointestinal tract, and poor dietary choices are among the primary contributors to Leaky Gut Syndrome. A diet rich in processed foods, high in refined sugars, and low in fiber can fuel inflammation within the gut. Gluten and dairy products, in particular, have been implicated in causing gut irritation and may contribute to the breakdown of the intestinal barrier.

Chronic Stress:

The mind-body connection is a potent force, and chronic stress can significantly impact gut health. Stress triggers the release of hormones such as cortisol, which can influence the permeability of the gut lining. Prolonged periods of stress may compromise the tight junctions between epithelial cells, potentially leading to Leaky Gut.

Medications:

Certain medications, though necessary for managing various health conditions, can inadvertently contribute to Leaky Gut Syndrome. Nonsteroidal anti-inflammatory drugs (NSAIDs) and antibiotics, for example, can disrupt the balance of gut bacteria, creating an environment conducive to increased permeability. Balancing the therapeutic benefits of medications with their potential impact on gut health is a crucial consideration in managing and preventing Leaky Gut.

Environmental Factors:

The environment we live in, including exposure to toxins and pollutants, can influence gut health. Environmental toxins and certain food additives may contribute to inflammation and compromise the gut lining. Pesticides and chemicals found in some processed foods have been linked to disruptions in the delicate balance of the gut microbiota, potentially playing a role in Leaky Gut Syndrome.

Imbalance in Gut Microbiota:

The gut is home to a vast community of microorganisms collectively known as the microbiota. Maintaining a healthy balance in this microbial ecosystem is essential for overall gut health. An imbalance in the gut microbiota, termed dysbiosis, can lead to inflammation and compromise the integrity of the gut lining. Factors such as overuse of antibiotics, a lack of dietary fiber, and exposure to environmental toxins can disrupt the equilibrium of the microbiota, potentially contributing to Leaky Gut.

Genetic Predisposition:

While lifestyle factors play a significant role in the development of Leaky Gut Syndrome, genetic predisposition also plays a role. Some individuals may have a genetic susceptibility to gut-related issues, making them more prone to disruptions in the gut barrier. Understanding one's genetic makeup can offer insights into potential vulnerabilities and inform personalized strategies for managing and preventing Leaky Gut.

Inflammatory Conditions:

Chronic inflammatory conditions, such as inflammatory bowel disease (IBD) and celiac disease, can contribute to the development of Leaky Gut Syndrome.

In these conditions, persistent inflammation in the gastrointestinal tract can damage the gut lining, compromising its integrity and leading to increased permeability. Managing the underlying inflammatory condition is essential in addressing and preventing Leaky Gut in these cases.

Lifestyle Factors:

Certain lifestyle choices can influence the risk of developing Leaky Gut. Smoking and excessive alcohol consumption, for example, have been associated with increased intestinal permeability. Adopting a lifestyle that prioritizes overall well-being, including regular exercise and adequate sleep, can positively impact gut health and reduce the risk of Leaky Gut Syndrome.

The causes and risk factors associated with Leaky Gut Syndrome are multifaceted, involving a combination of dietary, environmental, genetic, and lifestyle influences. Recognizing these factors empowers individuals to make informed choices that promote gut health and reduce the risk of developing or exacerbating Leaky Gut. A holistic approach, addressing both the underlying causes and symptoms, is key to restoring and maintaining a healthy balance within the intricate tapestry of the gastrointestinal system.

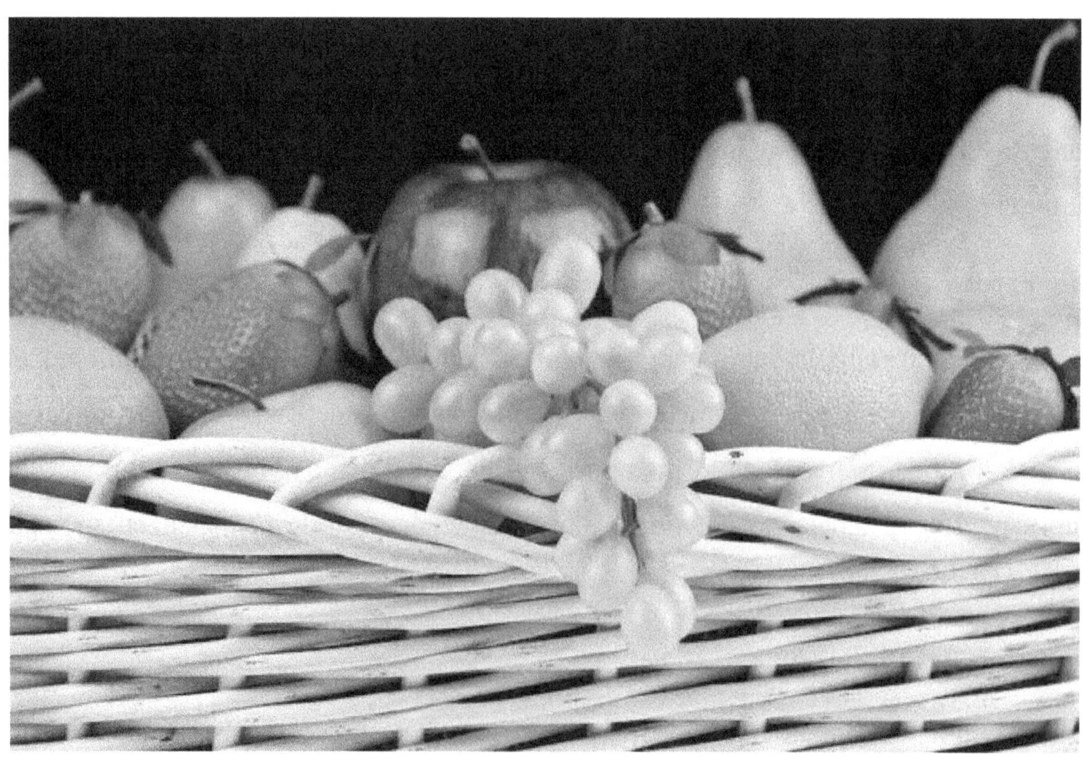

CHAPTER TWO

Symptoms and Diagnosis

Symptoms of Leaky Gut Syndrome are diverse and often nonspecific, making diagnosis a challenging task. The manifestations of this condition can extend beyond digestive distress, offering a complex tapestry of signals that warrant attention and investigation.

Digestive Distress:

Bloating, gas, diarrhea, and irritable bowel syndrome (IBS) are common symptoms associated with Leaky Gut. Individuals may experience fluctuations in bowel habits and find that their digestive system is more reactive to certain foods.

Food Sensitivities:

Leaky Gut often leads to the development of food sensitivities. Individuals may find that they react adversely to foods they previously tolerated well. This can manifest as allergic reactions, skin issues, or digestive discomfort upon consuming specific foods.

Joint Pain:

Inflammation triggered by Leaky Gut can extend beyond the digestive system, affecting joints and causing pain and stiffness. Joint pain may be particularly noticeable in individuals with autoimmune conditions linked to Leaky Gut.

Skin Conditions:

The skin serves as a visible reflection of internal health, and Leaky Gut can manifest in various skin conditions. Eczema, psoriasis, and other inflammatory skin conditions may be indicative of underlying gut issues.

Autoimmune Disorders:

Some researchers propose a connection between Leaky Gut Syndrome and autoimmune diseases. The immune system, triggered by substances leaking into the bloodstream, may become overactive and attack the body's own tissues, leading to autoimmune conditions.

Diagnosis Challenges:

Diagnosing Leaky Gut Syndrome is not straightforward due to the absence of a specific diagnostic test. Healthcare providers typically rely on a combination of medical history, symptoms, and exclusion of other conditions. Laboratory tests, including blood tests and stool analysis, may be utilized to assess inflammation and overall gut health.

Comprehensive Assessment:

Healthcare professionals often take a comprehensive approach to diagnosis, considering the individual's medical history, dietary habits, and lifestyle factors. Identifying patterns of symptoms and their correlation with potential triggers helps in the diagnostic process.

Laboratory Tests:

Blood tests may be employed to assess markers of inflammation and immune activity. Stool analysis can provide insights into the composition of the gut microbiota and identify any imbalances that may contribute to Leaky Gut.

Exclusion of Other Conditions:

Since the symptoms of Leaky Gut overlap with those of various gastrointestinal disorders, healthcare providers may need to rule out other conditions, such as inflammatory bowel disease (IBD) and celiac disease, through additional tests.

The symptoms of Leaky Gut Syndrome are varied and may present differently in each individual. Diagnosis requires a careful consideration of symptoms, medical history, and laboratory results to unravel the intricate web of factors contributing to this complex and often elusive condition.

Importance of a Healthy Microbiome

In the human body, an often-overlooked masterpiece unfolds within the realm of the gut — the microbiome. Comprising trillions of microorganisms, including bacteria, viruses, fungi, and other microbes, the microbiome is a complex tapestry that plays a crucial role in maintaining overall health. The importance of a healthy microbiome extends far beyond the confines of the digestive system, influencing diverse aspects of our well-being.

At the heart of this microscopic realm lies a delicate balance, a symbiotic dance between the host and its microbial inhabitants. This intricate balance is vital for the proper functioning of the digestive system, nutrient absorption, immune response, and even mental health. The microbiome acts as a dynamic ecosystem, constantly adapting to external influences, diet, and lifestyle choices.

One of the primary functions of a robust microbiome is its pivotal role in digestion. Microbes aid in the breakdown of complex carbohydrates, proteins, and fats that our body cannot digest alone. The byproducts of this digestive collaboration include essential nutrients and short-chain fatty acids, which are vital for energy production and the overall health of the gut lining. Without a diverse and well-balanced microbiome, the efficiency of this digestive process falters, potentially leading to nutrient deficiencies and compromised energy levels.

Beyond digestion, the microbiome acts as a formidable guardian of the immune system. The intricate interplay between the gut and the immune system is a fascinating testament to the microbiome's influence on our overall health. A healthy microbiome helps train and regulate the immune system, distinguishing between friend and foe. When this balance is disrupted, as seen in conditions like leaky gut syndrome, the immune system may misidentify harmless substances as threats, triggering unnecessary inflammatory responses.

In recent years, scientific research has uncovered the significant impact of the microbiome on mental health. The gut-brain axis, a bidirectional communication network between the gut and the brain, relies heavily on the microbiome as a mediator. Microbes produce neurotransmitters, such as serotonin and dopamine, which play a crucial role in regulating mood and emotional well-being. An imbalanced microbiome has been linked to mental health disorders, including anxiety and depression, highlighting the far-reaching consequences of neglecting the health of our microbial allies.

Maintaining a healthy weight is yet another facet of well-being influenced by the microbiome. Research suggests that the composition of the microbiome differs between individuals who are lean and those who struggle with obesity. A diverse microbiome appears to be associated with better metabolic health, aiding in weight regulation and reducing the risk of obesity-related complications. The intricate relationship between the microbiome and metabolism underscores the importance of nurturing this internal ecosystem for overall health.

In chronic diseases, the microbiome emerges as a potential player in prevention and management. Conditions such as inflammatory bowel disease (IBD), irritable bowel syndrome (IBS), and even autoimmune disorders have been linked to imbalances in the gut microbiome. Understanding and harnessing the therapeutic potential of the microbiome has become a focal point in medical research, paving the way for innovative interventions that target the root cause of various health challenges.

Nutrition plays a pivotal role. A diet rich in fiber, fermented foods, and prebiotics provides the necessary nourishment for a diverse microbial community. Fiber serves as the fuel for beneficial bacteria, promoting their growth and activity. Fermented foods, such as yogurt, kefir, and sauerkraut, introduce beneficial live cultures into the gut, enhancing microbial diversity. Prebiotics, found in foods like garlic, onions, and bananas, act as the fertilizer for these friendly microbes, ensuring their continued flourishing.

In addition to dietary considerations, lifestyle factors also significantly impact the microbiome. Antibiotic use, stress, lack of physical activity, and environmental exposures can disrupt the delicate balance of the microbiome. Mindful choices, such as reducing unnecessary antibiotic use, managing stress through practices like meditation, engaging in regular exercise, and minimizing exposure to environmental toxins, contribute to the overall well-being of the microbiome.

As we navigate the complexities of modern life, acknowledging the importance of a healthy microbiome becomes paramount. It is a dynamic ally, intricately woven into the fabric of our well-being, influencing everything from digestion to mental health. Embracing a holistic approach that encompasses mindful nutrition, lifestyle choices, and a deep understanding of the symbiotic relationship between the host and its microbial companions empowers us to cultivate and cherish this internal masterpiece. In doing so, we embark on a journey towards vibrant health, where the intricacies of the microbiome contribute to the harmonious symphony of our overall well-being.

Impact of Diet on Gut Health

In the intricate world of human physiology, the impact of diet on gut health emerges as a central and influential force. The choices we make in the realm of nutrition reverberate through the delicate ecosystem of the gut, shaping its composition and function.

Beyond mere sustenance, our dietary habits play a pivotal role in either nurturing a flourishing garden of beneficial microbes or paving the way for disruption and imbalance within the intricate tapestry of the gut microbiome.

The Foundations of Gut Health

To comprehend the impact of diet on gut health, one must first acknowledge the symbiotic relationship between the foods we consume and the microbial inhabitants of our digestive system. The gut microbiome, a diverse community of bacteria, viruses, fungi, and other microorganisms, thrives on a diet rich in fiber, prebiotics, and essential nutrients. This intricate interplay forms the foundation of a healthy gut ecosystem, where a harmonious balance fosters optimal digestion, nutrient absorption, and immune function.

Inflammatory Foods and Gut Disarray

In the complex choreography of the gut, certain dietary choices can disrupt the delicate balance and lead to inflammation. Highly processed foods laden with artificial additives, sugars, and unhealthy fats can act as catalysts for gut disarray.

These inflammatory foods not only compromise the integrity of the gut lining but also provide an environment conducive to the proliferation of harmful bacteria. The resulting imbalance may contribute to conditions such as leaky gut syndrome, where the intestinal barrier becomes permeable, allowing toxins to enter the bloodstream and triggering inflammatory responses.

Gut-Friendly Foods:

Conversely, a diet rich in gut-friendly foods serves as a cornerstone for cultivating and maintaining a thriving microbiome. Whole, plant-based foods, abundant in fiber, promote the growth of beneficial bacteria. Fiber acts as a prebiotic, a substance that fuels the growth and activity of these friendly microbes. Fruits, vegetables, whole grains, and legumes offer a diverse array of nutrients that support both the host and its microbial allies. Antioxidants, vitamins, and minerals found in these foods contribute not only to overall health but also to the resilience of the gut ecosystem.

The Role of Probiotics:

In the intricate dance of diet and gut health, probiotics emerge as key players. Probiotics are live microorganisms, predominantly beneficial bacteria, that confer health benefits when consumed in adequate amounts. Fermented foods, such as yogurt, kefir, sauerkraut, and kimchi, serve as rich sources of naturally occurring probiotics. By incorporating these foods into our diet, we introduce beneficial microbes into the gut, enhancing its microbial diversity and reinforcing the population of friendly bacteria.

Balancing Act:

Beyond digestion and immunity, the impact of diet on gut health extends to weight management. The composition of the gut microbiome has been linked to metabolic health and body weight. Research suggests that individuals with a more diverse microbiome may be better equipped to regulate weight and resist obesity-related complications. Therefore, mindful dietary choices that foster microbial diversity contribute not only to gut health but also to overall metabolic well-being.

Navigating the Modern Dietary Landscape

In the modern dietary landscape, where processed foods and convenience often take precedence, intentional choices become paramount for maintaining a healthy gut. Reading food labels, prioritizing whole foods, and minimizing the consumption of artificial additives and sugars are steps toward nurturing gut health. Adopting a predominantly plant-based diet, rich in a variety of colorful fruits and vegetables, ensures a broad spectrum of nutrients that support both human and microbial cells.

Mind-Gut Connection:

The intricate relationship between diet and gut health extends beyond the physical aspects of well-being to impact mental health. The gut-brain axis, a bidirectional communication network between the gut and the central nervous system, highlights the profound connection between our digestive system and emotional well-being. Emerging research suggests that the gut microbiome can influence mood and cognitive function, emphasizing the importance of a nourishing diet in promoting mental health.

Leaky Gut foods to eat and avoid

A condition known as Leaky Gut Syndrome unravels, disrupting the delicate balance of the digestive system.

Characterized by increased intestinal permeability, this condition allows undigested food particles, toxins, and bacteria to escape from the gut into the bloodstream, triggering immune responses and inflammation.

Understanding the role of diet in managing Leaky Gut becomes paramount, as certain foods can either exacerbate or alleviate the symptoms. Navigating this dietary terrain involves a careful selection of foods to eat and a deliberate avoidance of those that contribute to gut permeability.

Foods to Embrace:

Bone Broth: Rich in collagen and amino acids, bone broth provides essential building blocks for repairing the intestinal lining. It also supports the growth of beneficial gut bacteria, fostering a healthier microbial environment.

Fermented Foods: Probiotic-rich foods like yogurt, kefir, sauerkraut, and kimchi introduce beneficial bacteria into the gut. These microbes contribute to the restoration of a balanced microbiome and aid in the digestion process.

Omega-3 Fatty Acids: Found in fatty fish, flaxseeds, and walnuts, omega-3 fatty acids possess anti-inflammatory properties. Incorporating these foods helps reduce inflammation in the gut, potentially alleviating symptoms of Leaky Gut Syndrome.

Coconut Products: Coconut oil and coconut products contain medium-chain triglycerides (MCTs) with antimicrobial properties. These can support gut health by combating harmful bacteria while promoting the growth of beneficial ones.

Colorful Vegetables: Non-starchy vegetables like leafy greens, broccoli, and bell peppers are rich in fiber, antioxidants, and vitamins. They contribute to a diverse and nourishing diet that supports overall gut health.

Bone Broth: Rich in collagen and amino acids, bone broth provides essential building blocks for repairing the intestinal lining. It also supports the growth of beneficial gut bacteria, fostering a healthier microbial environment.

Ginger and Turmeric: These anti-inflammatory spices can be beneficial for individuals with Leaky Gut Syndrome. Incorporating ginger and turmeric into meals or consuming them as teas may help reduce inflammation in the gut.

Foods to Limit or Avoid:

Gluten-Containing Grains: Wheat, barley, and rye contain gluten, a protein that can contribute to gut inflammation and permeability. Removing or limiting gluten from the diet is often recommended for individuals with Leaky Gut Syndrome.

Dairy Products: Some individuals with Leaky Gut may experience sensitivity to dairy products. Lactose and casein, present in milk and dairy, can be problematic for those with compromised gut health. Opting for dairy alternatives or selecting lactose-free options may be advisable.

Processed Foods: High in additives, preservatives, and refined sugars, processed foods can contribute to inflammation and disrupt the balance of gut bacteria. Choosing whole, unprocessed foods is crucial for supporting gut health.

High Sugar and Artificial Sweeteners: Excessive sugar consumption and artificial sweeteners can negatively impact gut health by promoting the growth of harmful bacteria. Choosing natural sweeteners in moderation, such as honey or maple syrup, may be a better alternative.

Alcohol: Alcohol can irritate the intestinal lining and disrupt the gut microbiome. Limiting or avoiding alcohol is often recommended for individuals with Leaky Gut Syndrome to support the healing process.

Caffeine: Excessive caffeine intake can be a potential irritant to the gut lining. While moderate consumption may be tolerated, individuals with Leaky Gut Syndrome may benefit from reducing their caffeine intake or opting for less acidic alternatives.

Nightshade Vegetables: Some individuals may experience sensitivity to nightshade vegetables like tomatoes, peppers, and eggplants. These vegetables contain compounds that can contribute to inflammation, and eliminating or reducing their consumption may be beneficial for some individuals.

Personalized Approach and Professional Guidance

It's essential to recognize that individual responses to foods can vary, and there is no one-size-fits-all approach to managing Leaky Gut Syndrome through diet. A personalized approach, tailored to an individual's specific sensitivities and needs, is often crucial.

Seeking guidance from healthcare professionals, such as a registered dietitian or functional medicine practitioner, can provide valuable insights into crafting a suitable dietary plan.

Gut Health Principles and Guidelines

In the complex web of human health, the principles and guidelines governing gut health stand as pillars supporting overall well-being. A thriving gut ecosystem plays a pivotal role in digestion, nutrient absorption, immune function, and even mental health. Nurturing this intricate system involves embracing key principles and guidelines that foster a balanced and resilient gut environment.

1. Diverse and Plant-Rich Diet:

At the heart of gut health lies the diversity and quality of one's diet. A plant-rich diet, encompassing a variety of fruits, vegetables, whole grains, and legumes, provides an array of fibers, vitamins, and antioxidants that support microbial diversity.

A diverse microbiome is associated with improved digestion, enhanced nutrient absorption, and a more robust immune system. Including a rainbow of colorful plant foods in daily meals nourishes the gut microbiota, contributing to a flourishing ecosystem.

2. Fiber as a Foundation: Building Gut Resilience:

Fiber serves as the cornerstone of a gut-friendly diet. Found in fruits, vegetables, whole grains, and legumes, fiber is the preferred fuel for beneficial gut bacteria. As these microbes ferment fiber, they produce short-chain fatty acids, which contribute to gut health by nourishing the cells lining the intestines. Adequate fiber intake promotes regular bowel movements, prevents constipation, and supports the overall health of the gastrointestinal tract.

3. Probiotics for Gut Harmony:

Probiotics are live microorganisms, mainly beneficial bacteria, that confer health benefits when consumed in sufficient quantities. Incorporating probiotic-rich foods into the diet, such as yogurt, kefir, sauerkraut, kimchi, and other fermented foods, introduces beneficial microbes to the gut. These probiotics contribute to the balance of the microbiome, aiding in digestion, immune function, and the prevention of harmful bacterial overgrowth.

4. Prebiotics as Microbial Fuel:

Prebiotics are non-digestible fibers found in certain foods that serve as fuel for beneficial gut bacteria. Foods rich in prebiotics include garlic, onions, leeks, asparagus, bananas, and whole grains. By consuming prebiotic-rich foods, individuals provide the necessary substrates for the growth and activity of beneficial bacteria, promoting a healthy and balanced microbiome.

5. Hydration for Digestive Vitality:

Adequate hydration is fundamental to overall health and plays a crucial role in supporting digestive function. Water helps maintain the mucosal lining of the intestines, facilitates the movement of food through the digestive tract, and aids in the absorption of nutrients. Staying well-hydrated is a simple yet effective way to promote gut health and prevent issues such as constipation.

6. Mindful Eating Practices:

Mindful eating involves paying attention to the sensory experience of eating, being aware of hunger and fullness cues, and savoring each bite. This practice extends beyond nutrition; it has implications for gut health. Stress and rushed eating can negatively impact digestion, leading to issues such as bloating and discomfort. By adopting mindful eating habits, individuals support the digestive process and promote a harmonious relationship between the mind and the gut.

7. Limiting Inflammatory Foods:

Certain foods can contribute to inflammation and disrupt the delicate balance of the gut microbiome. Highly processed foods, sugary snacks, and those containing artificial additives may promote the growth of harmful bacteria while diminishing the population of beneficial microbes. Limiting or avoiding these inflammatory foods helps create an environment conducive to gut health, reducing the risk of conditions like Leaky Gut Syndrome.

8. Moderating Alcohol and Caffeine:

While moderate alcohol consumption and caffeine intake can be part of a healthy lifestyle for many, excessive consumption may negatively impact gut health. Alcohol can irritate the intestinal lining, and high caffeine intake may disrupt the gut-brain axis. Moderation in the consumption of these substances supports gut balance and overall well-being.

9. Individualized Approaches:

It's crucial to acknowledge that each individual's gut microbiome is unique, shaped by genetics, environment, and lifestyle. What works well for one person may not be optimal for another. Tailoring dietary choices to individual preferences, tolerances, and sensitivities allows for a personalized approach to gut health. Understanding one's bioindividuality empowers individuals to make informed decisions that align with their specific needs.

10. Seeking Professional Guidance:

For those facing specific gut health challenges or seeking to optimize their digestive well-being, seeking professional guidance is invaluable. Registered dietitians, nutritionists, and healthcare practitioners specializing in gut health can provide personalized recommendations based on individual health histories and goals. Professional guidance ensures that dietary choices align with overall health objectives and contribute to the restoration and maintenance of a resilient gut ecosystem.

In following the gut healthy diet squarely, adherence to these principles and guidelines forms the basis for a holistic approach to well-being. The intricacies of the gut microbiome demand thoughtful consideration, and by embracing these principles, individuals weave a tapestry of habits that nurtures a thriving gut environment.

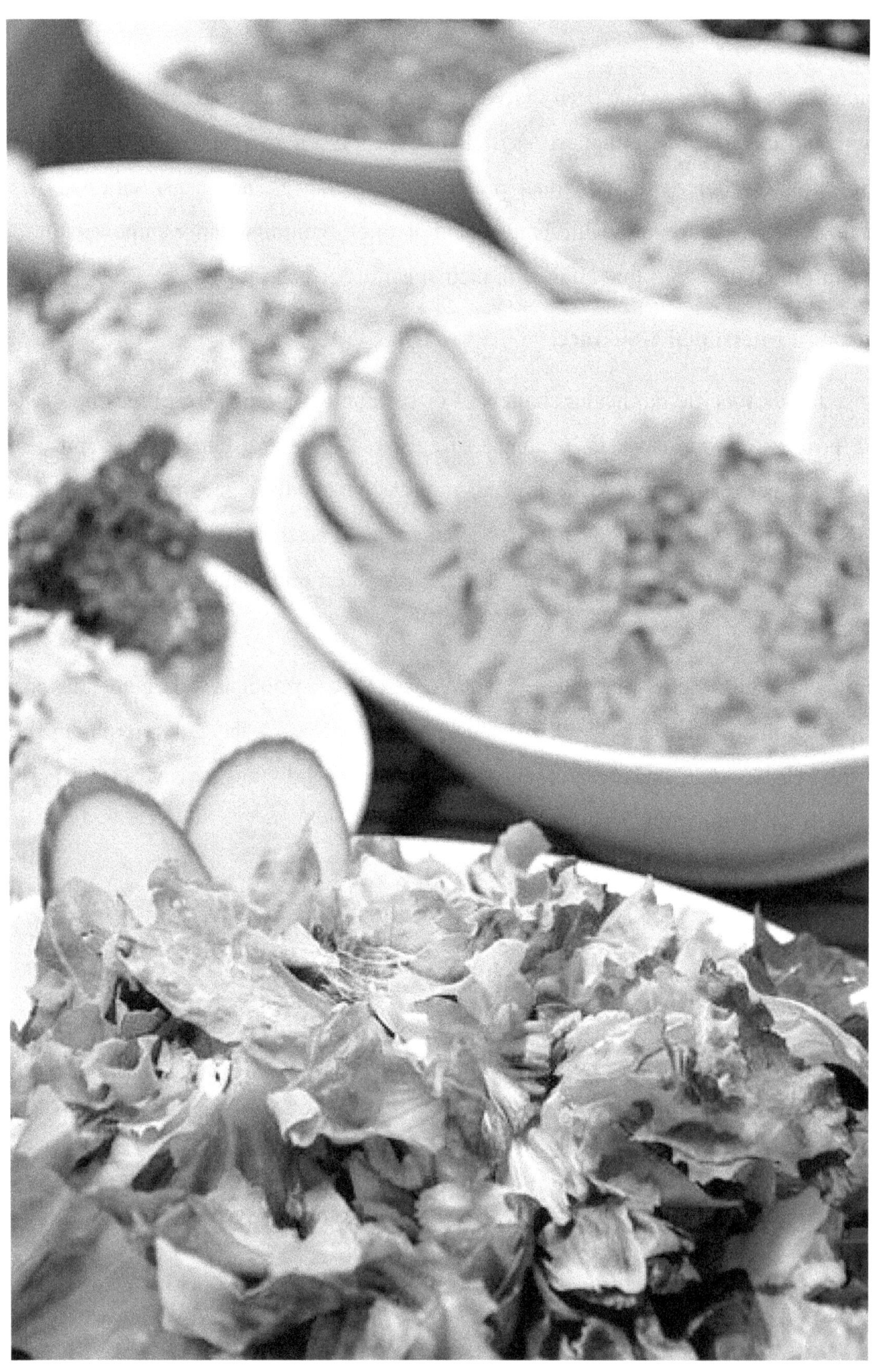

CHAPTER THREE

Healthy Leaky Gut Friendly Recipes

Breakfast Recipes

1. Healing Green Smoothie Bowl

Ingredients:

1 cup spinach leaves

1/2 cucumber, peeled and sliced

1/2 avocado

1/2 cup fresh pineapple chunks

1 tablespoon chia seeds

1 cup coconut water

Instructions:

Blend spinach, cucumber, avocado, pineapple, chia seeds, and coconut water until smooth.

Pour into a bowl and top with sliced berries and a sprinkle of pumpkin seeds.

Preparation Time: 10 minutes

2. Quinoa Porridge with Berries

Ingredients:

1/2 cup quinoa, rinsed

1 cup almond milk

1/2 teaspoon cinnamon

1/4 teaspoon ginger powder

1/2 cup mixed berries (blueberries, raspberries)

Instructions:

In a saucepan, combine quinoa, almond milk, cinnamon, and ginger.

Bring to a boil, then reduce heat and simmer until quinoa is cooked and mixture thickens.

Top with mixed berries and a drizzle of honey.

Preparation Time: 15 minutes

3. Gut-Healing Chia Pudding

Ingredients:

3 tablespoons chia seeds

1 cup coconut milk

1/2 teaspoon vanilla extract

1/2 cup sliced kiwi

1 tablespoon shredded coconut

Instructions:

Mix chia seeds, coconut milk, and vanilla extract in a jar. Stir well and refrigerate overnight.

In the morning, layer chia pudding with sliced kiwi in a glass.

Top with shredded coconut.

Preparation Time: 5 minutes (plus overnight chilling)

4. Turmeric and Ginger Infused Oatmeal

Ingredients:

1/2 cup gluten-free rolled oats

1 cup water or almond milk

1/2 teaspoon ground turmeric

1/4 teaspoon grated ginger

1 tablespoon maple syrup

1/4 cup sliced strawberries

Instructions:

Cook oats with water or almond milk, turmeric, and ginger until creamy.

Sweeten with maple syrup and top with sliced strawberries.

Preparation Time: 10 minutes

5. Coconut Flour Pancakes

Ingredients:

1/4 cup coconut flour

2 eggs

1/2 cup coconut milk

1/2 teaspoon baking soda

1/4 teaspoon vanilla extract

Fresh berries for topping

Instructions:

Mix coconut flour, eggs, coconut milk, baking soda, and vanilla extract until smooth.

Cook small pancakes on a griddle or pan.

Serve with fresh berries on top.

Preparation Time: 15 minutes

6. Gut-Friendly Acai Bowl

Ingredients:

1 pack unsweetened frozen acai

1/2 banana

1/2 cup unsweetened almond milk

Toppings: gluten-free granola, sliced kiwi, and a drizzle of honey

Instructions:

Blend frozen acai, banana, and almond milk until smooth.

Pour into a bowl and top with granola, sliced kiwi, and honey.

Preparation Time: 5 minutes

7. Sweet Potato and Kale Hash

Ingredients:

1 sweet potato, diced

1 cup kale, chopped

1 tablespoon olive oil

2 eggs

Salt and pepper to taste

Instructions:

Sauté sweet potato and kale in olive oil until cooked.

Push vegetables to the side and crack eggs into the pan, cooking to your preference.

Season with salt and pepper.

Preparation Time: 20 minutes

8. Probiotic-Rich Yogurt Parfait

Ingredients:

1 cup coconut yogurt

1/4 cup gluten-free granola

1/2 cup mixed berries

1 tablespoon chia seeds

Instructions:

Layer coconut yogurt with granola, mixed berries, and chia seeds.

Repeat layers as desired.

Preparation Time: 5 minutes

9. Spinach and Tomato Omelette

Ingredients:

2 eggs

1/2 cup baby spinach

1/4 cup cherry tomatoes, sliced

1 tablespoon olive oil

Salt and pepper to taste

Instructions:

Whisk eggs and pour into a heated pan with olive oil.

Add spinach and tomatoes, folding the omelette over.

Season with salt and pepper.

Preparation Time: 10 minutes

10. Blueberry and Almond Butter Smoothie

Ingredients:

1 cup blueberries

1 tablespoon almond butter

1/2 cup almond milk

1/2 banana

1 scoop collagen powder (optional)

Instructions:

Blend blueberries, almond butter, almond milk, banana, and collagen powder until smooth.

Pour into a glass and enjoy.

Preparation Time: 5 minutes

11. Cinnamon Baked Apples

Ingredients:

2 apples, cored and sliced

1/2 teaspoon cinnamon

1 tablespoon coconut oil

1/4 cup chopped walnuts

Instructions:

Toss apple slices with cinnamon and coconut oil.

Bake until apples are tender, then top with chopped walnuts.

Preparation Time: 20 minutes

12. Buckwheat Banana Pancakes

Ingredients:

1/2 cup buckwheat flour

1/2 ripe banana, mashed

1/2 cup almond milk

1/2 teaspoon baking powder

Fresh berries for topping

Instructions:

Mix buckwheat flour, mashed banana, almond milk, and baking powder until smooth.

Cook small pancakes on a griddle or pan.

Top with fresh berries.

Preparation Time: 15 minutes

13. Gut-Healing Matcha Latte

Ingredients:

1 teaspoon matcha powder

1 cup almond milk

1/2 teaspoon honey

Optional: Collagen powder or gut-friendly protein powder

Instructions:

Whisk matcha powder into a small amount of hot water to form a paste.

Heat almond milk and mix with matcha paste.

Sweeten with honey and add collagen or protein powder if desired.

Preparation Time: 5 minutes

14. Zucchini and Carrot Muffins

Ingredients:

1 cup grated zucchini

1/2 cup grated carrot

2 eggs

1/4 cup coconut flour

1/4 cup almond flour

1/2 teaspoon baking soda

Instructions:

Mix grated zucchini, carrot, eggs, coconut flour, almond flour, and baking soda.

Spoon into muffin cups and bake until golden.

Preparation Time: 25 minutes

15. Chia Seed Breakfast Pudding

Ingredients:

3 tablespoons chia seeds

1 cup coconut milk

1/2 teaspoon vanilla extract

Toppings: Sliced strawberries, chopped nuts, and a drizzle of honey

Instructions:

Mix chia seeds, coconut milk, and vanilla extract in a jar. Stir well and refrigerate overnight.

In the morning, layer chia pudding with sliced strawberries and top with chopped nuts and honey.

Preparation Time: 5 minutes (plus overnight chilling)

Lunch Recipes

1. Quinoa and Vegetable Buddha Bowl

Ingredients:

1 cup cooked quinoa

1 cup mixed vegetables (broccoli, bell peppers, carrots)

1/2 cup shredded kale

1/4 cup sliced avocado

2 tablespoons olive oil

1 tablespoon lemon juice

Salt and pepper to taste

Instructions:

In a pan, sauté mixed vegetables in olive oil until tender.

Assemble the bowl with quinoa, sautéed vegetables, shredded kale, and sliced avocado.

Drizzle with lemon juice and season with salt and pepper.

Preparation Time: 20 minutes

2. Salmon and Sweet Potato Patties

Ingredients:

1 can (14 oz) canned salmon, drained

1 cup mashed sweet potatoes

1/4 cup almond flour

1 egg

1 teaspoon lemon zest

1/2 teaspoon garlic powder

Salt and pepper to taste

Instructions:

In a bowl, combine salmon, mashed sweet potatoes, almond flour, egg, lemon zest, garlic powder, salt, and pepper.

Form mixture into patties and cook in a skillet until golden brown on each side.

Preparation Time: 25 minutes

3. Turkey and Vegetable Stir-Fry

Ingredients:

1 pound ground turkey

2 cups mixed stir-fry vegetables (broccoli, snap peas, bell peppers)

2 tablespoons coconut oil

2 tablespoons tamari (gluten-free soy sauce)

1 tablespoon ginger, minced

2 cloves garlic, minced

Instructions:

In a skillet, cook ground turkey in coconut oil until browned.

Add mixed vegetables, ginger, and garlic. Stir-fry until vegetables are tender.

Add tamari and toss until well combined.

Preparation Time: 20 minutes

4. Zucchini Noodles with Pesto and Cherry Tomatoes

Ingredients:

2 medium zucchinis, spiralized

1 cup cherry tomatoes, halved

1/4 cup pine nuts

1/2 cup fresh basil leaves

1/4 cup nutritional yeast

2 cloves garlic

1/3 cup olive oil

Salt and pepper to taste

Instructions:

Spiralize zucchinis and set aside.

In a food processor, blend pine nuts, basil, nutritional yeast, garlic, and olive oil to make pesto.

Toss zucchini noodles with pesto and cherry tomatoes. Season with salt and pepper.

Preparation Time: 15 minutes

5. Chicken and Vegetable Lettuce Wraps

Ingredients:

1 pound ground chicken

1 cup mixed vegetables (water chestnuts, carrots, mushrooms)

2 tablespoons coconut aminos

1 tablespoon sesame oil

Butter lettuce leaves for wrapping

Instructions:

In a skillet, cook ground chicken until browned.

Add mixed vegetables, coconut aminos, and sesame oil. Cook until vegetables are tender.

Spoon the mixture into lettuce leaves to create wraps.

Preparation Time: 20 minutes

6. Cauliflower Fried Rice with Shrimp

Ingredients:

1 head cauliflower, grated

1 pound shrimp, peeled and deveined

1 cup mixed vegetables (peas, carrots, corn)

2 eggs, beaten

2 tablespoons coconut oil

2 tablespoons gluten-free soy sauce

Instructions:

In a pan, sauté shrimp in coconut oil until cooked. Remove and set aside.

Add grated cauliflower and mixed vegetables to the pan, stir-frying until tender.

Push the cauliflower mixture to the side, pour beaten eggs into the pan, and scramble.

Combine shrimp, scrambled eggs, and cauliflower mixture. Stir in soy sauce.

Preparation Time: 30 minutes

7. Spinach and Turkey Stuffed Bell Peppers

Ingredients:

4 bell peppers, halved

1 pound ground turkey

1 cup spinach, chopped

1/2 cup quinoa, cooked

1 can (14 oz) diced tomatoes, drained

1 teaspoon Italian seasoning

Salt and pepper to taste

Instructions:

Preheat the oven to 375°F (190°C).

In a skillet, cook ground turkey until browned. Add chopped spinach and cook until wilted.

In a bowl, combine cooked turkey, quinoa, diced tomatoes, Italian seasoning, salt, and pepper.

Fill bell pepper halves with the turkey mixture. Bake for 25-30 minutes.

Preparation Time: 40 minutes

8. Gut-Healing Chicken Soup

Ingredients:

1 pound boneless, skinless chicken thighs

1 onion, chopped

2 carrots, sliced

2 celery stalks, chopped

3 cloves garlic, minced

8 cups chicken broth (preferably homemade)

1 teaspoon turmeric powder

1 teaspoon ginger, grated

Salt and pepper to taste

Fresh parsley for garnish

Instructions:

In a large pot, combine chicken thighs, chopped onion, sliced carrots, chopped celery, minced garlic, chicken broth, turmeric, and grated ginger.

Bring to a boil, then reduce heat and simmer until chicken is cooked through.

Shred the chicken and season the soup with salt and pepper. Garnish with fresh parsley.

Preparation Time: 1 hour

9. Grilled Lemon Herb Salmon

Ingredients:

4 salmon fillets

2 tablespoons olive oil

2 tablespoons fresh lemon juice

1 teaspoon fresh thyme, chopped

1 teaspoon fresh rosemary, chopped

Salt and pepper to taste

Instructions:

Preheat the grill to medium-high heat.

In a bowl, mix olive oil, lemon juice, chopped thyme, chopped rosemary, salt, and pepper.

Brush the salmon fillets with the marinade and grill for 4-5 minutes on each side.

Preparation Time: 15 minutes

10. Avocado and Chicken Salad

Ingredients:

2 cups cooked chicken, shredded

2 avocados, diced

1 cup cherry tomatoes, halved

1/4 cup red onion, finely chopped

1/4 cup cilantro, chopped

2 tablespoons lime juice

Salt and pepper to taste

Lettuce leaves for serving

Instructions:

In a bowl, combine shredded chicken, diced avocados, cherry tomatoes, red onion, and cilantro.

Drizzle with lime juice and toss to combine. Season with salt and pepper.

Serve the salad in lettuce leaves.

Preparation Time: 20 minutes

11. Roasted Vegetable Quinoa Bowl

Ingredients:

1 cup quinoa, cooked

2 cups mixed vegetables (zucchini, cherry tomatoes, red onion)

2 tablespoons olive oil

1 teaspoon dried oregano

1 teaspoon smoked paprika

Salt and pepper to taste

1/4 cup feta cheese, crumbled

Instructions:

Preheat the oven to 400°F (200°C).

Toss mixed vegetables with olive oil, dried oregano, smoked paprika, salt, and pepper.

Roast vegetables in the oven for 20-25 minutes.

Assemble the bowl with cooked quinoa, roasted vegetables, and crumbled feta cheese.

Preparation Time: 30 minutes

12. Turkey and Vegetable Skewers

Ingredients:

1 pound turkey breast, cut into cubes

2 bell peppers, cut into chunks

1 zucchini, sliced

1 red onion, cut into wedges

2 tablespoons olive oil

1 teaspoon cumin

1 teaspoon smoked paprika

Salt and pepper to taste

Instructions:

Preheat the grill or grill pan.

In a bowl, mix turkey cubes, bell pepper chunks, zucchini slices, red onion wedges, olive oil, cumin, smoked paprika, salt, and pepper.

Thread the turkey and vegetables onto skewers.

Grill skewers for 10-12 minutes, turning occasionally.

Preparation Time: 25 minutes

13. Sweet Potato and Chicken Hash

Ingredients:

2 sweet potatoes, diced

1 pound chicken thighs, boneless and skinless, diced

1 onion, chopped

2 tablespoons coconut oil

1 teaspoon smoked paprika

1 teaspoon garlic powder

Salt and pepper to taste

Fresh parsley for garnish

Instructions:

In a skillet, heat coconut oil over medium heat.

Add diced sweet potatoes and cook until slightly tender.

Add diced chicken, chopped onion, smoked paprika, garlic powder, salt, and pepper. Cook until chicken is cooked through and sweet potatoes are golden.

Garnish with fresh parsley before serving.

Preparation Time: 30 minutes

14. Cauliflower and Broccoli Soup

Ingredients:

1 head cauliflower, chopped

2 cups broccoli florets

1 onion, chopped

3 cloves garlic, minced

4 cups vegetable broth

1/2 cup coconut milk

1 teaspoon turmeric powder

Salt and pepper to taste

Chives for garnish

Instructions:

In a pot, combine chopped cauliflower, broccoli florets, chopped onion, minced garlic, vegetable broth, coconut milk, turmeric powder, salt, and pepper.

Bring to a boil, then reduce heat and simmer until vegetables are tender.

Blend the soup until smooth using an immersion blender or a countertop blender.

Garnish with chives before serving.

Preparation Time: 40 minutes

15. Mediterranean Tuna Salad

Ingredients:

2 cans (5 oz each) tuna, drained

1 cucumber, diced

1 cup cherry tomatoes, halved

1/4 cup Kalamata olives, sliced

1/4 cup red onion, finely chopped

2 tablespoons olive oil

1 tablespoon red wine vinegar

1 teaspoon dried oregano

Salt and pepper to taste

Feta cheese for topping

Instructions:

In a bowl, combine drained tuna, diced cucumber, cherry tomatoes, sliced Kalamata olives, and chopped red onion.

In a small bowl, whisk together olive oil, red wine vinegar, dried oregano, salt, and pepper. Pour over the tuna mixture and toss to combine.

Top with crumbled feta cheese before serving.

Preparation Time: 15 minutes

Dinner recipes

1. Gut-Healing Chicken and Vegetable Stir-Fry

Ingredients:

1 lb boneless, skinless chicken breasts, thinly sliced

2 cups broccoli florets

1 bell pepper, thinly sliced

1 zucchini, thinly sliced

2 tablespoons coconut oil

2 tablespoons tamari (gluten-free soy sauce)

1 teaspoon grated ginger

2 cloves garlic, minced

Salt and pepper to taste

Instructions:

Heat coconut oil in a skillet over medium-high heat.

Add sliced chicken and cook until browned.

Add ginger and garlic, stir for a minute.

Add broccoli, bell pepper, and zucchini. Cook until vegetables are tender-crisp.

Pour tamari over the stir-fry, toss to combine.

Season with salt and pepper to taste.

Serve over quinoa or cauliflower rice.

Preparation Time: 30 minutes

2. Quinoa and Roasted Vegetable Buddha Bowl

Ingredients:

1 cup quinoa, cooked

1 sweet potato, cubed

1 cup cherry tomatoes, halved

1 cup baby spinach

1/4 cup pumpkin seeds

2 tablespoons olive oil

1 teaspoon cumin

Salt and pepper to taste

Lemon tahini dressing (optional)

Instructions:

Preheat oven to 400°F (200°C).

Toss sweet potato cubes and cherry tomatoes with olive oil, cumin, salt, and pepper.

Roast in the oven for 20-25 minutes until vegetables are tender.

Assemble bowls with cooked quinoa, roasted vegetables, baby spinach, and pumpkin seeds.

Drizzle with lemon tahini dressing if desired.

Preparation Time: 40 minutes

3. Salmon and Asparagus Foil Packets

Ingredients:

2 salmon fillets

1 bunch asparagus, trimmed

2 tablespoons olive oil

1 lemon, sliced

2 cloves garlic, minced

Fresh dill for garnish

Salt and pepper to taste

Instructions:

Preheat the oven to 400°F (200°C).

Place each salmon fillet on a piece of foil.

Arrange asparagus around the salmon.

Drizzle with olive oil, add minced garlic, and season with salt and pepper.

Place lemon slices on top.

Seal the foil packets and bake for 15-20 minutes until salmon is cooked.

Garnish with fresh dill before serving.

Preparation Time: 25 minutes

4. Gut-Healing Turkey and Vegetable Skillet

Ingredients:

1 lb ground turkey

1 onion, diced

2 carrots, grated

1 bell pepper, diced

1 zucchini, diced

1 cup spinach

2 tablespoons coconut oil

1 teaspoon turmeric

1 teaspoon cumin

Salt and pepper to taste

Instructions:

In a skillet, heat coconut oil over medium heat.

Add diced onion and cook until softened.

Add ground turkey, breaking it apart and cooking until browned.

Stir in turmeric and cumin.

Add grated carrots, diced bell pepper, and zucchini. Cook until vegetables are tender.

Add spinach and cook until wilted.

Season with salt and pepper to taste.

Preparation Time: 30 minutes

5. Gut-Friendly Veggie and Chicken Soup

Ingredients:

1 lb chicken breast, cooked and shredded

1 onion, diced

2 carrots, sliced

2 celery stalks, sliced

1 zucchini, diced

4 cups chicken broth (low sodium)

1 teaspoon turmeric

1 teaspoon ginger

Salt and pepper to taste

Fresh parsley for garnish

Instructions:

In a large pot, sauté diced onion until translucent.

Add sliced carrots, celery, and zucchini. Cook for a few minutes.

Pour in chicken broth and bring to a simmer.

Stir in shredded chicken, turmeric, and ginger.

Simmer until vegetables are tender.

Season with salt and pepper.

Garnish with fresh parsley before serving.

Preparation Time: 40 minutes

6. Gut-Healing Veggie and Turkey Stuffed Peppers

Ingredients:

4 bell peppers, halved and seeds removed

1 lb ground turkey

1 cup cauliflower rice

1 cup diced tomatoes

1 cup spinach, chopped

1 onion, diced

2 cloves garlic, minced

1 teaspoon oregano

1 teaspoon paprika

Salt and pepper to taste

Instructions:

Preheat the oven to 375°F (190°C).

In a skillet, cook ground turkey until browned.

Add diced onion and garlic, sauté until softened.

Stir in cauliflower rice, diced tomatoes, chopped spinach, oregano, paprika, salt, and pepper.

Fill halved bell peppers with the turkey mixture.

Bake in the oven for 25-30 minutes until peppers are tender.

Preparation Time: 45 minutes

7. Gut-Friendly Grilled Lemon Herb Chicken

Ingredients:

4 chicken breasts

1 lemon, juiced

2 tablespoons olive oil

2 cloves garlic, minced

1 teaspoon thyme

1 teaspoon rosemary

Salt and pepper to taste

Instructions:

In a bowl, mix lemon juice, olive oil, minced garlic, thyme, rosemary, salt, and pepper to create a marinade.

Place chicken breasts in the marinade and let sit for at least 30 minutes.

Preheat the grill to medium-high heat.

Grill chicken for 6-7 minutes per side or until cooked through.

Serve with a side of steamed vegetables or a gut-friendly salad.

Preparation Time: 40 minutes (including marination time)

8. Gut-Healing Zucchini Noodles with Pesto

Ingredients:

4 medium-sized zucchinis, spiralized

1 cup cherry tomatoes, halved

1/2 cup pine nuts

2 cups fresh basil leaves

1/2 cup extra-virgin olive oil

2 cloves garlic

1/4 cup nutritional yeast (optional)

Salt and pepper to taste

Instructions:

In a food processor, combine basil, pine nuts, garlic, and nutritional yeast (if using).

While blending, slowly add olive oil until a smooth pesto is formed.

In a large pan, sauté zucchini noodles until just tender.

Toss zucchini noodles with cherry tomatoes and pesto.

Season with salt and pepper to taste.

Preparation Time: 20 minutes

9. Gut-Friendly Turkey and Vegetable Skewers

Ingredients:

1 lb turkey breast, cut into cubes

1 zucchini, sliced

1 red onion, cut into chunks

1 bell pepper, cut into squares

2 tablespoons olive oil

1 teaspoon cumin

1 teaspoon paprika

Salt and pepper to taste

Instructions:

Preheat the grill or grill pan to medium-high heat.

In a bowl, mix turkey cubes with olive oil, cumin, paprika, salt, and pepper.

Thread turkey, zucchini slices, red onion chunks, and bell pepper squares onto skewers.

Grill for 10-12 minutes, turning occasionally, until turkey is cooked through.

Serve with a side of gut-friendly quinoa or cauliflower rice.

Preparation Time: 30 minutes

10. Gut-Healing Baked Cod with Lemon and Herbs

Ingredients:

4 cod fillets

1 lemon, sliced

2 tablespoons olive oil

2 tablespoons fresh parsley, chopped

1 teaspoon thyme

Salt and pepper to taste

Instructions:

Preheat the oven to 400°F (200°C).

Place cod fillets on a baking sheet lined with parchment paper.

Drizzle olive oil over the cod and season with thyme, salt, and pepper.

Arrange lemon slices on top of the fillets.

Bake for 15-20 minutes or until the fish is cooked through.

Garnish with chopped parsley before serving.

Preparation Time: 25 minutes

11. Gut-Friendly Vegetable and Lentil Soup

Ingredients:

1 cup dried green or brown lentils, rinsed

1 onion, diced

2 carrots, sliced

2 celery stalks, sliced

1 cup diced tomatoes

1 cup kale, chopped

4 cups vegetable broth (low sodium)

2 cloves garlic, minced

1 teaspoon turmeric

1 teaspoon cumin

Salt and pepper to taste

Instructions:

In a large pot, sauté diced onion until translucent.

Add sliced carrots, celery, and minced garlic. Cook for a few minutes.

Pour in vegetable broth and bring to a simmer.

Add lentils, diced tomatoes, turmeric, cumin, salt, and pepper.

Simmer until lentils are tender.

Stir in chopped kale and cook until wilted.

Preparation Time: 45 minutes

12. Gut-Healing Shrimp and Avocado Salad

Ingredients:

1 lb shrimp, peeled and deveined

2 avocados, diced

1 cucumber, sliced

1 cup cherry tomatoes, halved

1/4 cup red onion, finely chopped

2 tablespoons fresh cilantro, chopped

2 tablespoons olive oil

1 lime, juiced

Salt and pepper to taste

Instructions:

In a skillet, cook shrimp with olive oil until pink and opaque.

In a large bowl, combine diced avocados, sliced cucumber, cherry tomatoes, red onion, and cilantro.

Add cooked shrimp to the salad.

Drizzle with lime juice and olive oil.

Season with salt and pepper to taste.

Preparation Time: 20 minutes

13. Gut-Friendly Sweet Potato and Turkey Chili

Ingredients:

1 lb ground turkey

2 sweet potatoes, diced

1 can (15 oz) black beans, drained and rinsed

1 can (15 oz) diced tomatoes

1 bell pepper, diced

1 onion, diced

2 cloves garlic, minced

2 tablespoons chili powder

1 teaspoon cumin

Salt and pepper to taste

Instructions:

In a large pot, cook ground turkey until browned.

Add diced sweet potatoes, black beans, diced tomatoes, diced bell pepper, diced onion, and minced garlic.

Stir in chili powder and cumin.

Season with salt and pepper.

Simmer for 25-30 minutes until sweet potatoes are tender.

Preparation Time: 40 minutes

14. Gut-Healing Turkey and Kale Stuffed Acorn Squash

Ingredients:

2 acorn squash, halved and seeds removed

1 lb ground turkey

2 cups kale, chopped

1 onion, diced

2 cloves garlic, minced

1/4 cup dried cranberries (unsweetened)

2 tablespoons olive oil

1 teaspoon cinnamon

Salt and pepper to taste

Instructions:

Preheat the oven to 400°F (200°C).

Place acorn squash halves on a baking sheet.

In a skillet, cook ground turkey until browned.

Add chopped kale, diced onion, and minced garlic. Sauté until kale is wilted.

Stir in dried cranberries, olive oil, cinnamon, salt, and pepper.

Fill each acorn squash half with the turkey and kale mixture.

Bake for 25-30 minutes until squash is tender.

Preparation Time: 45 minutes

15. Gut-Friendly Eggplant and Turkey Lasagna

Ingredients:

1 lb ground turkey

1 eggplant, sliced lengthwise

1 cup spinach, chopped

1 can (15 oz) crushed tomatoes

1 onion, diced

2 cloves garlic, minced

2 tablespoons olive oil

1 teaspoon oregano

1 teaspoon basil

Salt and pepper to taste

Instructions:

Preheat the oven to 375°F (190°C).

In a skillet, cook ground turkey until browned.

Sauté diced onion and minced garlic until softened.

Add crushed tomatoes, oregano, basil, salt, and pepper. Simmer for 10 minutes.

In a separate pan, grill eggplant slices until tender.

In a baking dish, layer eggplant slices, turkey mixture, and chopped spinach.

Repeat the layers and finish with a layer of turkey mixture.

Bake for 30-35 minutes until bubbly and golden.

Preparation Time: 50 minutes

Snack Recipes

1. Avocado and Salmon Nori Rolls

Ingredients:

Nori sheets

Smoked salmon slices

Avocado, sliced

Cucumber, julienned

Sesame seeds

Coconut aminos (for dipping)

Instructions:

Place a nori sheet on a bamboo sushi rolling mat.

Layer smoked salmon, avocado, and cucumber along the nori sheet.

Roll tightly using the mat and seal the edge with a bit of water.

Slice into bite-sized pieces and sprinkle with sesame seeds.

Serve with coconut aminos for dipping.

Preparation Time: 15 minutes

2. Turmeric Roasted Almonds

Ingredients:

Raw almonds

Turmeric powder

Coconut oil

Sea salt

Instructions:

Toss almonds with melted coconut oil, turmeric, and a pinch of sea salt.

Spread evenly on a baking sheet.

Roast in the oven at 350°F (175°C) for 10-12 minutes.

Allow to cool before serving.

Preparation Time: 15 minutes

3. Coconut Yogurt Parfait

Ingredients:

Coconut yogurt

Fresh berries (blueberries, strawberries)

Chia seeds

Almond butter

Granola (gluten-free)

Instructions:

Layer coconut yogurt with fresh berries in a glass or bowl.

Drizzle with almond butter and sprinkle chia seeds.

Top with gluten-free granola.

Repeat layers as desired.

Preparation Time: 10 minutes

4. Baked Sweet Potato Chips

Ingredients:

Sweet potatoes, thinly sliced

Olive oil

Sea salt

Dried rosemary

Instructions:

Toss sweet potato slices with olive oil, sea salt, and dried rosemary.

Arrange in a single layer on a baking sheet.

Bake at 375°F (190°C) for 15-20 minutes until crispy.

Allow to cool before serving.

Preparation Time: 25 minutes

5. Gut-Healing Smoothie Bowl

Ingredients:

Frozen mixed berries

Spinach leaves

Banana

Chia seeds

Almond milk

Instructions:

Blend frozen berries, spinach, banana, and almond milk until smooth.

Pour into a bowl and top with chia seeds.

Preparation Time: 10 minutes

6. Cucumber and Hummus Bites

Ingredients:

Cucumber, sliced

Hummus

Cherry tomatoes, halved

Fresh parsley, chopped

Instructions:

Top cucumber slices with a small dollop of hummus.

Garnish with halved cherry tomatoes and fresh parsley.

Preparation Time: 10 minutes

7. Quinoa Salad Cups

Ingredients:

Cooked quinoa

Cherry tomatoes, diced

Cucumber, diced

Avocado, diced

Lemon juice

Fresh basil, chopped

Instructions:

Mix quinoa with diced tomatoes, cucumber, and avocado.

Drizzle with lemon juice and sprinkle fresh basil.

Spoon into small cups for easy serving.

Preparation Time: 15 minutes

8. Almond Butter and Banana Rice Cakes

Ingredients:

Rice cakes (gluten-free)

Almond butter

Banana, sliced

Chia seeds

Instructions:

Spread almond butter on rice cakes.

Top with banana slices and sprinkle chia seeds.

Preparation Time: 5 minutes

9. Mashed Avocado and Tomato on Rice Crackers

Ingredients:

Rice crackers (gluten-free)

Avocado, mashed

Cherry tomatoes, sliced

Sea salt and black pepper

Instructions:

Spread mashed avocado on rice crackers.

Top with sliced cherry tomatoes.

Season with sea salt and black pepper.

Preparation Time: 10 minutes

10. Roasted Red Pepper and Walnut Dip

Ingredients:

Roasted red peppers (jarred)

Walnuts

Garlic cloves

Olive oil

Lemon juice

Paprika

Instructions:

Blend roasted red peppers, walnuts, garlic, olive oil, and lemon juice until smooth.

Sprinkle with paprika before serving.

Preparation Time: 15 minutes

11. Zucchini Noodles with Pesto

Ingredients:

Zucchini, spiralized

Cherry tomatoes, halved

Pesto sauce (homemade or store-bought)

Pine nuts

Instructions:

Toss zucchini noodles with cherry tomatoes and pesto sauce.

Top with pine nuts before serving.

Preparation Time: 15 minutes

12. Berry and Coconut Chia Pudding

Ingredients:

Chia seeds

Coconut milk

Mixed berries (strawberries, blueberries)

Shredded coconut

Instructions:

Mix chia seeds with coconut milk and refrigerate for at least 2 hours or overnight.

Top with mixed berries and shredded coconut before serving.

Preparation Time: 5 minutes (plus chilling time)

13. Greek Salad Skewers

Ingredients:

Cherry tomatoes

Cucumber, diced

Feta cheese, cubed

Kalamata olives

Olive oil

Fresh oregano, chopped

Instructions:

Thread cherry tomatoes, cucumber, feta, and olives onto skewers.

Drizzle with olive oil and sprinkle with fresh oregano.

Preparation Time: 15 minutes

14. Seaweed and Cucumber Salad

Ingredients:

Seaweed salad mix

Cucumber, thinly sliced

Rice vinegar

Sesame oil

Sesame seeds

Instructions:

Mix seaweed salad with thinly sliced cucumber.

Dress with rice vinegar and sesame oil, then sprinkle sesame seeds.

Preparation Time: 10 minutes

15. Roasted Garlic and Rosemary White Bean Dip

Ingredients:

Cannellini beans, drained and rinsed

Roasted garlic cloves

Fresh rosemary, chopped

Lemon juice

Olive oil

Instructions:

Blend cannellini beans with roasted garlic, fresh rosemary, lemon juice, and olive oil until smooth.

Serve with vegetable sticks or gluten-free crackers.

Preparation Time: 20 minutes

CONCLUSION

In the exploration of recipes designed to support and nourish those grappling with Leaky Gut Syndrome, this cookbook endeavors to weave a tapestry of flavors, textures, and healing ingredients. Each recipe is crafted not merely for taste but with a keen understanding of the intricate relationship between gut health and overall well-being.

As we embark on this culinary journey, it is essential to recognize the profound impact of our dietary choices on the delicate ecosystem within. The principles of this cookbook, rooted in whole, nourishing foods and mindful preparation, serve as a guide to promoting gut resilience and restoration. The featured recipes aim not only to tantalize the taste buds but to provide a foundation for individuals seeking a path to digestive vitality.

In the realm of Leaky Gut, where the permeability of the intestinal lining presents a unique set of challenges, the recipes offered here emphasize ingredients known for their gut-healing properties. From bone broth that supports connective tissue repair to probiotic-rich foods that foster a diverse microbiome, each dish is a step towards reclaiming balance and fostering digestive wellness.

As we savor the flavors of these recipes, let us also acknowledge the significance of individualized approaches. Each person's journey to gut health is unique, influenced by factors such as genetics, lifestyle, and sensitivities. The recipes presented in this cookbook offer a foundation, but the art of crafting a leaky gut-friendly diet involves tailoring these recipes to one's specific needs and preferences.

Moreover, beyond the kitchen, the Leaky Gut Cookbook encourages a holistic approach to health. Mindful eating practices, stress management, and lifestyle choices complement the nourishing recipes within these pages. Together, they contribute to a comprehensive strategy for promoting not only gut health but overall vitality.

In closing, may this cookbook be a source of inspiration and empowerment on your journey towards digestive well-being. May the ingredients within these pages serve as allies in restoring harmony to the intricate dance of your gut. Embrace the flavors, savor the nourishment, and may your culinary adventures contribute to a healthier, more vibrant you. Cheers to a journey of healing through the artistry of mindful and purposeful cooking!